The
Little Book of
Health

D0540295

Also by Dr Michael Spira:

Basic Health Education (with Vincent Irwin)
How to Lose Weight Without Really Dieting
The No-Diet Book
The 3D Diet
Understanding Menopause
Understanding Nutrition
Angina
The 12-Minute Weight-Loss Plan

Dr Spira has also been a contributor to:

Everyman's Encyclopedia
The British Medical Association Complete Family Health Encyclopedia

The
Little Book of
Health

Simple Steps to a
Longer, Healthier,
Happier Life

Dr Michael Spira

vie

THE LITTLE BOOK OF HEALTH

Vie Books is an imprint of Summersdale Publishers Ltd

Summersdale Publishers Ltd
46 West Street
Chichester
West Sussex
PO19 1RP
UK

www.summersdale.com

Printed and bound in Poland

ISBN: 978-1-78685-234-2

Substantial discounts on bulk quantities of Summersdale books are available to corporations, professional associations and other organisations. For details contact general enquiries: telephone: +44 (0) 1243 771107 or email: enquiries@summersdale.com.

About the Author

Dr Michael Spira (MB, BS, MRCS, LRCP) qualified as a doctor at London's St Bartholomew's Hospital. After initially specialising in eye surgery, he is now a GP and medical director at a leading group of medical clinics, the Smart Clinics, in Chelsea, London. He is also the lead physician at BUPA South Kensington.

Besides his many books and articles, Dr Spira has regularly featured as a guest on national TV and radio, including as a medical expert on BBC One's *Kilroy*, ITV's *GMTV* and ITV's *The Gloria Hunniford Show*.

Disclaimer

Every effort has been made to ensure that the information in this book is accurate and current at the time of publication. The author and the publisher cannot accept responsibility for any misuse or misunderstanding of any information contained herein, or any loss, damage or injury, be it health, financial or otherwise, suffered by any individual or group acting upon or relying on information contained herein. None of the views or suggestions in this book is intended to replace medical opinion from a doctor who is familiar with your particular circumstances. If you have concerns about your health, please seek professional advice in person.

The opinions expressed in this book are those of Dr Michael Spira. These opinions do not necessarily reflect those of BUPA.

Contents

Introduction

This book came about as a result of my work with thousands of clients at my central London clinic specialising in health assessments. Time and time again, I am asked to give a few simple lifestyle tips for a healthier and longer life.

Most of the tips are evidence based – that is to say, they are backed up by solid scientific research. A small minority, while not necessarily based on science, are either so self-evident or based on a wealth of anecdotal evidence that they merit inclusion.

There is some overlap between some tips. But, more interestingly, some tips seem to contradict each other – for example, 'Drink more coffee' and 'Drink less coffee'. These contradictions reflect the controversial aspects of some health advice. Another example is the debate about screening for prostate cancer. I meet many urologists and ask them the question. Some say yes, always screen, while others say no. (I am pleased to say that the majority say yes, which is the advice I give in this book.)

If some of the apparent contradictions prompt you to do your own research that may be a good thing. But a word of caution: Dr Google can be confusing and misleading!

While these tips cannot guarantee a long and healthy life, they will certainly increase your chances of achieving it. So when you celebrate your ninetieth birthday, perhaps you'd like to let me know – assuming, of course, that I'm still around too!

Eat five a day

The benefits of five portions a day of fruit and vegetables, which are good sources of **antioxidants**, are strongly supported by scientific evidence. The most important benefits are a reduced risk of cardiovascular disease (heart disease and stroke) and cancer.

For each serving of fruit and veg you eat every day, **up to five servings**, you reduce your risk of premature death by an average of 5 per cent. There is not much additional benefit in going above five servings.

Portion examples include:

- **Half a grapefruit**

- An apple
- A banana
- A pear
- An orange
- Two plums
- Two satsumas
- Seven strawberries
- 14 cherries
- 30 g dried fruit (e.g. sultanas or raisins)
- Three heaped tbsp cooked vegetables
- Two broccoli florets.

Potatoes don't count, while fruit juices and smoothies count as only one portion even if more than 150 ml is drunk.

You need a **balanced diet**, which means both fruit and vegetables. But remember that a lot of fruit (e.g. bananas, grapes and mangoes) is high in sugar. In fact, the sweeter the fruit, the more sugar it has. **So it's best to eat more veggies than fruit**.

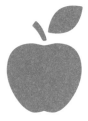

Watch the carbs

Don't ditch the carbs – you need them. But you need the *right* ones, as every carb has an effect on blood glucose (sugar) levels.

Sugar, potatoes, bread, pasta, most fruit, most cereals and short-grain rice all push up glucose levels fast and high. We call these high-GI (glycaemic index) carbs. You secrete more insulin when you eat these carbohydrates – and unfortunately insulin is great at promoting body fat, so you put on extra weight and your arteries get clogged up. In time, you may develop insulin resistance, which eventually tips over into type 2 diabetes. Plus you're more likely to develop coronary heart disease.

So what's the answer? Concentrate on low-GI carbs. Examples are apples, oranges, new potatoes, sweet potatoes, sourdough bread, small portions of wholemeal pasta cooked al dente, long-grain rice – these are good carbs.

A great resource for checking the GI index of your food is **glycemicindex.com**.

Healthy breakfast choices include:

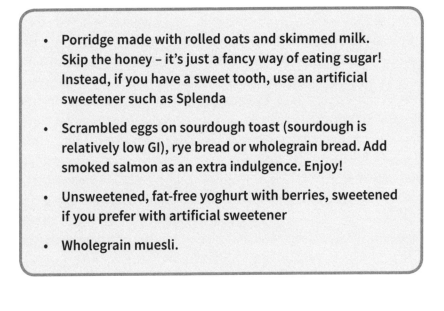

- **Porridge made with rolled oats and skimmed milk. Skip the honey – it's just a fancy way of eating sugar! Instead, if you have a sweet tooth, use an artificial sweetener such as Splenda**

- **Scrambled eggs on sourdough toast (sourdough is relatively low GI), rye bread or wholegrain bread. Add smoked salmon as an extra indulgence. Enjoy!**

- **Unsweetened, fat-free yoghurt with berries, sweetened if you prefer with artificial sweetener**

- **Wholegrain muesli.**

Eat more protein

Proteins are the **building blocks** of life. Every single one of your cells contains protein. You need protein in your diet in order to help your body repair cells, make new cells and to maintain your immune system.

Protein is vital for all of us but especially for the **growth** and **development** of children, teenagers and pregnant women. Men should aim for around 56 g per day, and women for 45 g.

The basic structure of protein is a chain of amino acids. Animal sources of amino acids include meat, fish, milk and eggs. Low-fat or skimmed milk is an excellent source of protein. Vegetarian sources include soy, beans, legumes, peanut butter and some grains, e.g. wheatgerm and quinoa.

Each ounce (roughly 30 g) of most protein-rich foods – including meat, poultry or fish – contains 7 g of protein.

The following amounts of these foods also contain approximately 7 g of protein:

- **1 large egg**
- **½ cup tofu**
- **½ cup lentils**
- **½ cup cooked beans**
- **1 tbsp (15 g) peanut butter.**

Bonus for slimmers!

Protein foods are slimmers' friends. This is because protein makes you feel fuller for longer, and it curbs carb highs and lows by slowing down the absorption of sugar from your stomach into the bloodstream.

Eat fewer saturated fats

Eating too much saturated fat may increase your levels of bad, low-density lipoprotein (LDL) cholesterol. This is the stuff that clogs up your arteries and can lead to **heart disease** and **strokes**.

Saturated fat is found in **fatty** and **processed** foods. These include meats such as sausage and bacon, plus full-fat dairy products, e.g. cheese, cream, butter, lard and ghee (a clarified butter found in South Asian and Arabic cooking).

Pies, pastries, cakes and biscuits contain saturated fats too. They're also in coconut oil and palm oil.

Over the page are some ways to cut back on saturated fats:

- **Chips:** use thick, straight-cut chips instead of French fries or crinkle-cut. At home, cook them in the oven with a little sunflower oil instead of deep-frying

- **Butter:** replace butter with a vegetable low-fat spread that has 0 g trans fats (unhealthy fatty acids) in general, and in recipes which call for butter, e.g. mashed potatoes

- **Milk:** use skimmed milk or soy/rice/hemp/almond milk instead of whole or semi-skimmed milk

- **Meat:** trim the visible fat off meat such as steak

- **Bacon:** use back bacon instead of streaky bacon, and grill rather than fry

- **Cheese:** use a strong-tasting cheese, such as mature Cheddar, to flavour a dish or sauce, as a little will go further

- **Yoghurt:** use low-fat or fat-free, sugar-free yoghurt

- **Pizza: choose a lower-fat topping – e.g. vegetables, ham or prawns – instead of pepperoni, salami or extra cheese.**

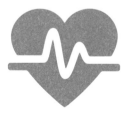

Take omega-3 supplements

Omega-3 fatty acids are a group of polyunsaturated fatty acids that are important for several body functions. Natural sources include oily fish, shellfish and some vegetable oils. If your diet is deficient in these, omega-3 supplements may be helpful, even though their benefits are not as proven as those of naturally occurring omega-3. You could also try incorporating **omega-3-fortified foods**, such as soy milk and yoghurt, into your diet.

Reasons omega-3 may boost your health:

- **Research suggests that omega-3s may help protect against Alzheimer's disease and dementia**

- **Omega-3 supplements can lower raised levels of triglycerides, a blood fat (high levels of which increase the risk of heart disease)**

- **Omega-3 oils can help lower levels of depression and reduce stiffness in rheumatoid arthritis sufferers.**

Caution: check with your doctor before using omega-3 supplements if you are:

- **Pregnant, trying to become pregnant or breastfeeding**

- **Taking medicine that affects blood clotting**

- **Allergic to fish or shellfish**

- **Considering giving a child an omega-3 supplement.**

Eat oatmeal for breakfast

Scientific evidence shows that eating oatmeal has many health benefits:

- It may lower LDL ('bad') cholesterol and reduce the risk of heart disease

- Oatmeal may reduce the risk of type 2 diabetes because oatmeal contains soluble fibre, which helps control blood glucose levels. The American Diabetes Association recommends oats for people with diabetes

- It may help you to lose or control your weight. This is because its soluble fibre absorbs water, which slows down your digestive process. This makes you feel fuller for longer

- **Oatmeal may help to reduce high blood pressure. Once again, this seems to be linked to the soluble fibre**

- **As well as being a good source of protein, complex carbohydrates and iron, oatmeal contains many vitamins, minerals and antioxidants.**

Oatmeal is delicious and easy to incorporate into your diet. Mix rolled oats with skimmed, semi-skimmed or soy milk and/or water and cook in a microwave for just a few minutes, then, if you like, add a few raisins or berries. Alternatively, you could make your own muesli with oats, dried fruit plus a variety of seeds and nuts.

URBAN MYTH:
It's unhealthy to miss breakfast

To miss breakfast or not? That is the question.

The issue is whether or not people who miss breakfast are more likely to become overweight or obese. The evidence suggests that you don't catch up on the calories you skip at breakfast, but instead compensate by preserving energy, e.g. you use the lift or fidget less at your desk, which results in fewer calories being burned.

A study published in 2014 in *The American Journal of Clinical Nutrition* showed that in a controlled trial of 283 people, there was **no difference in weight gain** between those who ate breakfast and those who didn't.

Ultimately it comes down to what works best for you and what's most comfortable. If you're hungry first thing in the morning, then have a healthy breakfast. But if you're not hungry, and especially if you're overweight, it's perfectly OK to skip breakfast.

By the way, this doesn't necessarily apply to schoolchildren. If they miss breakfast and then feel hungry mid-morning, they probably won't have the opportunity to eat until it's time for their school lunch. So encourage children to have a healthy breakfast – if that means a cereal, ensure it's low in sugar content.

Eat more oily fish

Doctors became interested in the health benefits of oily fish (e.g. salmon, sardines and mackerel) when they realised that oily-fish-eating Eskimos have fewer heart attacks and strokes than other peoples. They discovered that this is because oily fish are rich in omega-3 fatty acids as well as vitamin D, selenium, some B vitamins and protein.

The most important benefit, and one that has been proved by science, is the **reduced risk of cardiovascular disease** (heart disease and strokes). Ideally you should eat two portions of fish a week, at least one of which should be oily.

Other possible benefits, for which the scientific evidence isn't quite so strong, include a reduced risk of prostate cancer, dementia, rheumatoid arthritis and blindness due to macular degeneration.

Eat less red and processed meat

Yes, red meat – beef, lamb, pork, etc. – is a great source of **protein** and of **iron**. But too much isn't good for you.

A high consumption of red meat and processed meat gives you too much saturated fat, which leads to an increase in artery-clogging cholesterol – a major factor in coronary heart disease.

But there's another reason why you should go easy with red meat. Over the past few years, a definite link has been found between excessive red-meat consumption and bowel cancer.

A safe amount of red meat is **up to three portions a week**. A portion is 120 g (4 oz) – that's a thin slice the size of the palm of your hand.

Eat more fibre

Fibre is an important part of a healthy balanced diet. It can help prevent many health problems, including:

- **Heart disease, by reducing bad cholesterol**
- **Some cancers, especially colon (large bowel) cancer**
- **Type 2 diabetes**
- **Overweight and obesity.**

Fibre is found only in foods from **plants**, such as beans, grains, vegetables and fruit. There are two types of fibre – **soluble and insoluble** – both of which are beneficial.

Sources of **soluble** fibre include:

- **Oats, barley and rye**
- **Fruit, e.g. apples and bananas**
- **Root vegetables, e.g. potatoes and carrots.**

Sources of **insoluble** fibre include:

- **Bran**
- **Cereals**
- **Wholemeal bread**
- **Nuts and seeds.**

Eating high-fibre foods will help you feel fuller for longer. This may be useful if you are trying to lose weight.

If you need to increase your fibre intake, it's important to do so **gradually**, as a sudden increase may make you produce more wind and feel bloated, and can give you stomach cramps. If you are increasing your fibre, make sure you drink plenty of **fluids**.

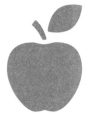

Eat blueberries

Blueberries are a good source of vitamin K, vitamin C, fibre, manganese and several other antioxidants, especially anthocyanin.

Research shows that women who eat at least three portions of blueberries a week have a 32 per cent lower risk of a heart attack compared with those who eat blueberries once a month or less. However, the study could not prove that this fruit definitely caused the lower risk.

Research suggests that blueberries may reduce the risk of atherosclerosis, the condition of the arteries that can lead to heart attacks and strokes.

The other great thing about blueberries is that they are **very low in calories** – there are fewer than 100 calories in a full cup.

Great ways to eat blueberries

- Added to breakfast cereal or oatmeal

- Mixed with low-fat yoghurt to make a delicious low-calorie dessert

- Blended into a healthy smoothie.

Eat smaller portions

The **more** you eat, especially in a single meal, the **higher** your blood sugar levels rise. And higher blood sugar levels lead to more insulin being secreted by your pancreas. Insulin not only reduces blood sugar levels – it also promotes body fat. This makes it difficult to lose or control your weight.

Another consequence of high insulin levels is that, over time, your body may become **resistant to insulin**. This in turn can lead to type 2 diabetes and all the unhealthy consequences of that disease.

Scientific studies have shown that people who eat **smaller portions** – and therefore fewer calories – live **longer, healthier lives**.

Consider intermittent fasting

Intermittent fasting has several health benefits, including:

- **Helping to reduce weight and body fat, especially abdominal fat, which in turn leads to:**

- **Improved blood sugar levels, leading to a reduction of insulin resistance (prediabetes), which in turn leads to:**

- **Reducing the risk of type 2 diabetes**

- **Reducing several risk factors, including LDL ('bad') cholesterol, triglycerides (a group of blood fats) and inflammatory markers (substances produced in the body as a result of inflammation)**

- **Possibly reducing the risk of various cancers and Alzheimer's**
- **Possibly increasing lifespan.**

There are many different ways of doing intermittent fasting – find the one that suits your lifestyle.

Popular methods of intermittent fasting include:
- Reducing your calorie intake to no more than 500 a day on two days per week
- Reducing your calorie intake to around 750 a day on alternate days
- Eating just once a day every day.

Of course, there are many variations on the above. All the options, including the once-a-day eating, are surprisingly easy to get used to for most people.

Eat more chocolate

Yes, I know this is contrary to much of the advice out there. After all, most chocolate contains a lot of sugar and fat. But studies have shown that **dark chocolate** – chocolate with at least 70 per cent cocoa – can **improve health** and **lower the risk of heart disease**.

A study of nearly 20,000 people showed that those who ate an average of 6 g (0.2 oz) of dark chocolate per day had a 39 per cent lower risk of heart attack or stroke.

Dark chocolate is a great source of antioxidants. It can improve blood flow and lower blood pressure. Plus it increases blood levels of HDL cholesterol – that's the good, protective cholesterol we all need. Dark chocolate may also protect your skin from sun damage and improve brain function.

But it must be **dark** chocolate – chocolate that is mainly cocoa. And you should eat it **in moderation** because in addition to its good nutritional content, it still contains calories.

Moderation is about two or three small squares of a typical chocolate bar.

A great exercise tip

Eat six to eight small squares of a plain chocolate bar before and during your workout. Dark chocolate contains nitrates that boost endurance and recovery from sport. Nitrates are converted to nitric oxide in the body, which dilates blood vessels and reduces oxygen consumption. This allows you to go further for longer.

Artificial sweeteners cause cancer

This is one of the most common myths to be found on the internet. It all started many, many years ago, when a few laboratory beagle dogs developed tumours after being fed saccharine at doses equivalent to a gazillion times those humans eat. Well, what should we believe?

Artificial sweeteners are regulated in the United States by the Food and Drug Administration (FDA), one of the world's toughest food and drug regulatory authorities. In a word, the FDA's take on sweeteners is that they are perfectly *safe*. According to the FDA (and other authorities), there are **no significant risks** associated with sweeteners despite them being 'artificial'.

Another world-recognised authority on scientific matters is the National Library of Medicine in Washington, which has millions of scientifically validated online articles. A search through those articles shows that the possibility of artificial sweeteners causing cancer is **negligible**. The European Food Safety Authority (EFSA), another tough regulatory body, also considers sweeteners **safe**.

The evidence says that it's safe for you to use artificial sweeteners to help manage your weight, but remember that substituting sweeteners for added sugar plays only a small part in weight control. You need to watch those carbs and fats – and take plenty of exercise.

Have a glass of red wine with dinner

If you're confused by the conflicting messages in the media on alcohol's effects on health, you're not alone – even doctors aren't sure what to advise.

But now the picture is clearer. A meta-analysis (a statistical analysis that looks at data from multiple studies) in the highly regarded medical journal *Circulation* (published in March 2016) analysed the findings of 23 studies conducted on nearly 30,000 participants between 1966 and 2016, looking at the effects of alcohol on health.

The analysis showed that although there is consistent evidence that habitual, moderate alcohol intake can be beneficial, there is some evidence that there may be a transiently higher risk of heart attack and stroke immediately after drinking alcohol – even for smaller amounts (1 unit a day). The complex physiological effects of alcohol result in both higher and lower cardiovascular risk depending on the amount consumed and drinking frequency.

Alcohol consumption was associated with an immediately higher cardiovascular risk that was significantly reduced after 24 hours. In fact, within a day moderate alcohol intake was actually protective against heart attacks and haemorrhagic strokes, and protective against ischaemic strokes within one week. However, heavy alcohol drinking was associated with higher cardiovascular risk during the following day and week.

> The take-home message is: moderate alcohol consumption has health benefits, whereas heavy consumption is dangerous.

As regards red wine specifically, this contains an antioxidant called resveratrol, and there is some scientific evidence that this may help prevent cancer.

Restrict alcohol to no more than 14 units per week

How mean is **14 units** a week?! By many people's standards it doesn't sound a lot. Fourteen units is about 1½ bottles of wine, or 7 pints of lager or cider, or 14 single measures of spirits such as gin, vodka or whisky.

So 14 units a week is safe? Well, actually, no. There is no such thing as a safe limit. Although alcohol may taste wonderful – and, in small amounts, may make you feel good – it is a **poison**. Alcohol affects not only your liver, but your heart, brain, kidneys and blood pressure, and can increase the risk of several types of cancer: breast, mouth, throat and oesophagus (gullet). Fourteen units a week is considered 'low risk', but this is not the same as 'safe'.

It's important to avoid drinking a lot in one session. Binge drinking can increase the risk of injuries and accidents, such as head injuries and fractures, as well as alcohol poisoning and stomach haemorrhage.

Enjoy alcohol – but in moderation. Here are some tips to cut down your alcohol intake:

- **Before you start drinking, set a limit on how much you're going to drink**

- **Tell your family and friends you're cutting down and ask them to support you**

- **Have smaller drinks**

- **Have a drink with a lower alcohol content**

- **Keep hydrated. Drink plenty of water before you start drinking and quench your thirst with non-alcoholic drinks. One glass of water for every alcoholic drink is a good guideline to follow**

- **Have several alcohol-free days every week.**

Drink plenty of fluids

Many of us don't drink enough fluids and are therefore dehydrated. Apart from obviously feeling thirsty, a common but often unrecognised symptom of dehydration is tiredness.

In addition to thirst, the two signs of dehydration that are easiest to spot are producing dark-coloured, strong-smelling urine and passing urine less often than usual.

The internet is full of 'advice', such as drink at least eight glasses or 2 litres of water per day. But, frankly, who is measuring? And is this even the right advice?

A simple and perfectly accurate way of ensuring an adequate fluid intake is to drink enough so that you don't ever feel thirsty. Passing pale urine is a good clue that you're well hydrated.

Remember to increase your fluids:

- **When exercising**
- **During hot weather**
- **If you have diarrhoea.**

Don't eat late at night

Avoid late-night eating – that is, eating 1.5–2 hours before your bedtime.

Reasons to avoid eating late:

- It disturbs your body clock and melatonin levels, so that your body reacts differently to food
- The *British Journal of Obesity* showed (in 2015) that people who ate later experienced a dip in their metabolic rate, with a reduced ability to burn off carbs
- It can increase the number of times you need to visit the lavatory during the night.

High-fat and **spicy** foods are more likely to make you feel full and disturb your sleep. If, for whatever reason, you can't avoid eating late, try to eat only **healthy foods**, e.g. vegetables, sourdough bread and raw nuts.

Other good choices are foods that contain **tryptophan**, an amino acid that can help induce relaxation and sleep, such as turkey, dairy products, bananas and almonds.

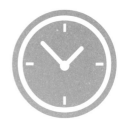

Cut back on salt

We all need some salt – to help control blood pressure and for nerves and muscles to work properly.

But too much salt (more than 5 g per day) isn't good for you. It can lead to **high blood pressure**, which in turn can lead to:

- **Stroke**
- **Heart failure**
- **Kidney failure.**

Here are some ways to cut your salt intake:

- Use less salt when cooking and at the table

- Add flavour with herbs, spices or pepper instead of salt

- Eat fewer processed foods

- Read the labels to see how much salt is in bought food.

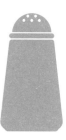

Take a vitamin D supplement each day

Vitamin D is known as the 'sunshine vitamin' because sunshine is the main source of this important vitamin. However, 50 per cent of the worldwide population and 85 per cent of the UK population is deficient in this vitamin. It is one of the few supplements I routinely advise my patients to take.

Most people know about the link between vitamin D deficiency and bone disease. But many other health problems arise from a lack of this vitamin. These include cancer, heart disease, fractures and falls, type 2 diabetes, depression, dementia, infectious diseases such as flu, and much more. A recent study showed that people who are vitamin D deficient are more prone to headaches.

Unless you are able to expose yourself to at least 20 minutes of sunshine every day, I recommend a dose of 25 mcg (1,000 IU [International Unit]) daily.

Consider taking calcium supplements

Calcium is the most common mineral in your body. It is important for:

- **Building strong bones and teeth**
- **Regulating muscle contractions, including the heartbeat**
- **Blood clotting.**

In children a lack of calcium can cause the bone disease rickets. Too little calcium in older adults can cause osteoporosis (the thinning of bones).

Good food sources of calcium include:

- **Dairy foods, such as milk and cheese**

- **Green leafy vegetables, e.g. broccoli, okra, kale and cabbage (but not spinach)**

- **Bread and anything made with fortified flour**

- **Fish where you eat the bones, e.g. sardines and pilchards**

- **Tofu**

- **Nuts**

- **Soya beans**

- **Soya drinks with added calcium.**

Adults need 700 mg of calcium a day. If your diet doesn't incorporate plenty of the above calcium-rich foods, then consider taking a calcium supplement. I usually recommend a daily calcium supplement of 1,500 mg. This dose is perfectly safe, but don't take more (too much can increase the risk of coronary heart disease).

Consider taking magnesium supplements

Magnesium is a mineral that:

- Helps turn the food you eat into energy
- Is important for bone health
- Is needed for muscle and nerve function
- Is necessary for normal heart rhythm.

Good food sources of magnesium include:

- Green leafy vegetables, e.g. spinach and kale
- Legumes
- Nuts
- Seeds
- Wholegrains
- Foods fortified with magnesium, e.g. some breakfast cereals.

For good levels of magnesium, follow a diet which includes:

- **A variety of vegetables, fruit and wholegrains**
- **Skimmed or semi-skimmed milk, milk products and oils**

- **A variety of protein foods, including seafood, lean meats and poultry, eggs, legumes (beans and peas), nuts, seeds and soy products.**

The following people need a magnesium supplement:

- People with gastrointestinal diseases
- People with type 2 diabetes
- Alcoholics
- Older adults, especially those over 70.

If your diet isn't a healthy, balanced one, and for whatever reason you can't (or choose not to) improve it, or if you belong to one of the four groups above, consider a magnesium supplement – **400 mg** daily.

Consider taking folic acid

Folic acid is a B vitamin we all need to make red blood cells. A deficiency can cause anaemia – when you don't have enough red blood cells or haemoglobin (the part of your red blood cells that carries oxygen) to meet your body's oxygen needs. Apart from preventing anaemia and spinal cord defects in the foetus (for which reason all pregnant women are advised to take folic acid supplements before and during the first 12 weeks of pregnancy), there is some evidence that extra folic acid *may* help prevent coronary heart disease and strokes.

Folic acid (or folate) is found naturally in a wide variety of foods. It is also present in foods fortified with folic acid. Vegetables are a good source of folic acid, but if the veggies are overcooked much of the vitamin is destroyed.

Good natural sources of folic acid include:

- **Spinach, broccoli, cabbage, Brussels sprouts and kale**
- **Beans and legumes**
- **Oranges**
- **Wheat bran and wholegrain foods**
- **Poultry, liver, pork, shellfish**
- **Yeast and beef extracts**
- **Fortified foods, e.g. some breakfast cereals.**

A safe dose of folic acid supplement is **400 mcg**. Taking too much folic is unlikely to happen with natural foods, but there is a possibility that excessive folic acid supplements *may* increase the risk of bowel cancer, so never exceed a dose of 1,000 mcg.

Take turmeric

Turmeric is a spice that comes from the turmeric plant and is one of the main spices in curry. It contains the chemical **curcumin**, which has lots of rumoured health benefits.

The benefits of curcumin for which there is the most scientific evidence:

- **Reduces high cholesterol. Studies suggest that taking turmeric extract by mouth twice daily for three months reduces total cholesterol, LDL ('bad') cholesterol and triglycerides (another blood fat) in overweight people with high cholesterol**

- **Alleviates osteoarthritis ('wear and tear' arthritis).
  Studies show that turmeric extract can reduce pain and
  improve function in osteoarthritis sufferers.**

Other health problems which are said to benefit from turmeric, but
for which the evidence is not yet so convincing, include:

- **Dyspepsia (upset stomach)**

- **Crohn's disease and ulcerative colitis (types of
  inflammatory bowel disease)**

- **Irritable bowel syndrome (IBS)**

- **Bowel cancer**

- **Diabetes (prevention in people with prediabetes)**

- **Reduces the risk of heart attack following heart bypass surgery**

- **Prostate cancer**

- **Rheumatoid arthritis**

- **Systemic lupus erythematosus (SLE, an inflammatory disease)**

- **Uveitis (a serious inflammation of the eye)**

- **Alzheimer's disease**

- **Depression**

- **Aids recovery from surgery.**

You can either add turmeric to your food or take a daily supplement.

Take a probiotic

Probiotics are live bacteria and yeasts that are good for your health – they're often referred to as 'good bacteria'. Probiotics live in the bowel and help keep it healthy – their main benefits are to do with the bowel. Some people take probiotics to alleviate specific symptoms, while others take them daily to give their health a little boost.

Probiotics can help various conditions, including:

- **Infectious diarrhoea caused by bacteria, viruses or parasites**
- **Diarrhoea caused by antibiotics**
- **Irritable bowel syndrome (IBS)**

- **Inflammatory bowel disease (ulcerative colitis or Crohn's disease)**
- **Lactose intolerance.**

It's also a good idea to take a probiotic while you're taking a broad-spectrum antibiotic (such as augmentin or erythromycin) because antibiotics can destroy the bowel flora (the bacteria that live in your bowel).

There have been claims that probiotics can help vaginal conditions such as BV (bacterial vaginosis) and vaginal thrush, but there isn't any good scientific evidence for this. Similarly, claims for benefits in eczema are unscientific.

Probiotics occur naturally and are also available as food supplements.

Foods that contain naturally occurring probiotics include:

- Yoghurt and kefir
- Dark chocolate
- Soy milk and tempeh
- Kimchi, pickles and sauerkraut
- Miso soup
- Sourdough bread.

You need a probiotic that can survive the acidic conditions of the stomach – most probiotics don't survive.

Robust probiotic supplements include:

- **Symprove, a water-based liquid supplement that contains four strains of live and active bacteria (available online)**

- **VSL#3, which contains eight strains of beneficial live bacteria (also available online).**

Drink less coffee – maybe

The benefits and harmful effects of drinking coffee are controversial, with conflicting scientific studies on this topic.

Too much caffeine can make you feel irritable and light-headed. It can also result in anxiety, headaches, increased heart rate, stomach pains and dehydration. Plus many people find they don't sleep so well if they drink coffee within 6 hours of bedtime.

Too much unfiltered coffee (boiled or espresso) can cause higher cholesterol levels. But, unlike what was previously thought, caffeine doesn't seem to increase the risk of heart disease, except in a small minority of people with a specific gene mutation that slows down the breakdown of caffeine in the body.

Widely accepted benefits of coffee (in any form) include:

- **Reduced risk of neurological conditions, especially Alzheimer's and Parkinson's disease**

- **Reduced risk of type 2 diabetes (this benefit does not seem to be related to the caffeine in coffee)**

- **Reduced risk of heart failure, but only in those who drink no more than two cups a day.**

My advice is this: if you drink **more than four cups** of coffee a day, cut back. Otherwise, continue to enjoy your coffee. But make sure you're not drinking too many milk-rich coffees (e.g. cappuccinos and flat whites) as these are high in saturated fats and calories. However, see the next health tip…

Drink more coffee – maybe

Bowel cancer, otherwise known as colorectal cancer or colon cancer, is one of the most common cancers and a leading cause of death. Scientific studies have shown that drinking four or more cups of coffee a day **significantly reduces the risk**. If you don't like to drink much caffeine, the good news is that **decaffeinated coffee** seems to be just as beneficial in helping prevent bowel cancer.

Other benefits of drinking more coffee (either caffeinated or decaf) are reduced risk of developing type 2 diabetes and liver disease.

So **four cups** of caffeinated or decaffeinated coffee a day is good.

An exercise tip

Caffeine is a great legal way to boost exercise performance. An espresso 20 minutes before you exercise can produce a 6 per cent improvement in power output during endurance exercise such as swimming, cycling, rowing and marathon running.

Drink decaffeinated coffee

Many people enjoy drinking coffee but want to limit their caffeine intake. Decaffeinated coffee is an excellent alternative.

There are many benefits of drinking decaf because decaffeinated coffee:

- **Is likely to promote many of the health benefits of caffeinated coffee but without caffeine's side effects (e.g. headaches, nervousness and shaking)**

- **Contains lots of antioxidants**

- **May cause less gastrointestinal discomfort**

- **Lowers liver enzymes as effectively as caffeinated coffee**

- **Possibly reduces the risk of bowel cancer.**

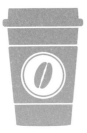

Drink more tea

Tea contains less caffeine than coffee, and herbal tea contains no caffeine at all. There are several health benefits of tea, some backed up with more reliable research than others:

- **Tea contains antioxidants called flavonoids**

- **Research suggests that tea may reduce LDL ('bad') cholesterol and the risk of heart disease and strokes**

- **Tea may help with weight loss. Research has shown that there is a correlation between tea consumption and lower BMI (body mass index) and lower waist circumference**

- Green tea (which contains less caffeine than black tea) may help protect your bones

- Tea may keep your smile bright by decreasing the erosion of tooth enamel. This seems to be due to changes in the pH (the acidity or alkalinity) in the mouth

- Tea may boost the immune system by tuning up immune cells so they reach their targets quicker

- Tea may help battle cancer, but there's no solid research on this

- Herbal teas, such as camomile and especially peppermint, seem to soothe the digestive system.

Sit less, stand more

It's long been known that it's healthier to stand than to sit for long periods, but why is standing good?

Many muscles in our legs, bottom and abdomen work in order to keep us standing. Since working muscles consume sugar and lower triglycerides (a group of blood fats), this in turn lowers cholesterol. Regularly standing reduces the risk of type 2 diabetes and heart disease.

If you must sit at work, try to stand up and walk around for 5 minutes every 20 minutes.

Do at least one hour of activity each day

A recent paper shows that **an hour** of moderate-intensity activity offsets the health risks of 8 hours of sitting.

A meta-analysis published in *The Lancet* showed that the health risks of sitting for 8 hours a day (including type 2 diabetes, cardiovascular disease, cancer and premature death) can be offset by 1 hour of moderate-intensity activity, which includes brisk walking (at 5.6 km/h) or cycling for pleasure (at 16 km/h). The research analysed data from 16 studies, with data on more than one million individuals aged 45 or older from the United States, Western Europe and Australia.

As well as the hour a day of physical activity, it's important to break up periods of sitting with **short bursts of activity**, such as walking for 5 minutes every 20 minutes.

Exercise with no pain is no good

We've all heard the saying 'Feel the burn', but is this really what you should be aiming for when you work out? And what exactly is the 'burn'?

The burn comes when there's a build-up of **lactic acid** in your muscles. Lactic acid is produced when you exercise at an intensity high enough to exhaust the muscles' supply of **oxygen**. Muscles need oxygen to break down the glucose that produces energy. If there's no oxygen, muscles use enzymes to break down the glucose, and lactic acid results. As the amount of lactic acid increases in your blood, you start to feel the 'burn'. This is an inevitable and acceptable consequence of high-intensity exercise.

It turns out that the maxim 'No pain, no gain' is not true. Burn and pain are not the same. Burn indicates muscle fatigue, while pain indicates that **injury** is about to happen or may already be happening. There is **nothing to be gained** by experiencing pain. In fact, if you feel pain while working out, and especially if you go past that point, there's a significant risk of injury.

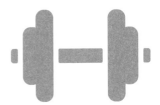

10,000 steps a day

Walking 10,000 steps a day can improve your health, build stamina and burn excess calories, but does the concept of 10,000 daily steps have any scientific basis?

This particular figure derives from Japan, where pedometers sold in the run-up to the 1964 Tokyo Olympics were marketed under the name *manpo-kei*, which translates to '10,000 steps meter'. While there's no scientific basis to the number 10,000, there certainly are benefits to walking several thousand steps per day.

One study found that women who increased their steps to nearly 10,000 a day reduced their blood pressure after 24 weeks. In another, overweight women who walked 10,000 steps a day improved their blood glucose levels.

Typically, for someone weighing around 70 kg, briskly walking 10,000 steps would burn around 400 kcal.

Ways to incorporate 10,000 steps into your day:

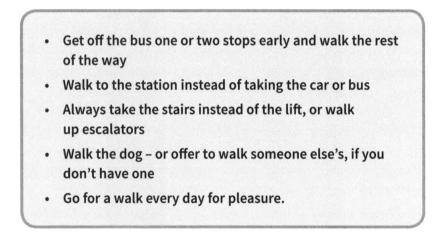

- **Get off the bus one or two stops early and walk the rest of the way**
- **Walk to the station instead of taking the car or bus**
- **Always take the stairs instead of the lift, or walk up escalators**
- **Walk the dog – or offer to walk someone else's, if you don't have one**
- **Go for a walk every day for pleasure.**

Remember that it's less important to focus on the number 10,000 than to simply **take as many steps as you can** every day, e.g. 8,000 daily steps will bring about very good health benefits.

HIIT – a shortcut to exercise?

One hundred and fifty minutes of moderate-level activity a week is often recommended, but it's sometimes hard to find the time for that. Hence HIIT, **high-intensity interval training**. HIIT is brief, intense and infrequent exercise.

A recent experiment looked at the effects of five bursts of intense exercise lasting 60 seconds, alternated with five 90-second relaxation intervals, done three times a week. Volunteers who did HIIT improved their VO2 max (maximal oxygen consumption, a measure of aerobic physical fitness) by 17 per cent, which is an enormous improvement and compares with a typical 12 per cent improvement in volunteers who did the conventional 150-minutes-a-week moderate exercise.

HIIT can either be **incorporated** into your usual exercise routine or simply **swapped** for it.

Do hand grips

In 2013 a landmark paper was published in *Hypertension*, an authoritative journal of the American Heart Association. The paper demonstrated that while all exercise was good for blood pressure, some of the most impressive improvements came after four weeks of hand-grip squeezing.

Inexpensive hand grippers can be bought online. If you prefer, you can use a rubber ball.

Squeeze the gripper or ball for 2 minutes at a time, for around 12–15 minutes, three times a week. Typically, you can expect a 10 per cent improvement in blood pressure, which will in turn reduce your risk of strokes.

If you have blood pressure greater than 130/80, this may be an excellent way of controlling it.

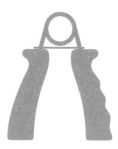

Lift with your legs, not your back

Back injuries are among the most common form of injury – and such injuries are almost always avoidable. Most are caused by incorrect lifting, usually over a period of time.

Lifting from your legs gives you the power and stability you need to move weight without hurting your back.

When you lift something heavy, bend your **knees** and **hips**, not your waist, before you grasp the object you're lifting, and with your back straight simply **stand up**. Your legs and hips are much stronger than your lower back. This way, you use your strength in your upper leg muscles and avoid unnecessary strain on the lower back.

You should also hold the object **close to your chest** to decrease the strain on the spine, and tighten your abdominal muscles. **Tightening**

your abs will hold your back in a good lifting position and will prevent putting excessive force on the spine.

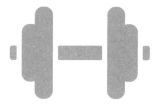

URBAN MYTH:
Crunches are the best way to flat abs

Although crunches help to tone abdominal muscles, reducing your waistline is much more about reducing body fat. The most effective exercises to achieve this involve your **entire core** – exercises which include your shoulders and buttocks.

Planks and **bridges** are the way to go. These are isometric core-strength exercises where you maintain a position similar to a push-up for the maximum time possible. These core exercises are a great and safe way to strengthen not only your abs but also your lower back and even your shoulders.

Have more sex

Besides being fun, science has shown that sex offers plenty of **health benefits**:

- **Sex is exercise – and exercise is good for the heart. Having sex twice a week or more reduces the risk of heart attack by half compared with those who have sex less than once a month**

- **Close body contact with someone you're fond of helps to lower blood pressure and reduces heart rate (you can also get this benefit from hugging a good friend)**

- **Sex is a great stress buster**

- **Regular sex boosts the immune system, which means that you're less likely to get infections**

- **Sex makes most people feel healthier**

- **Regular sex reduces the risk of stomach ulcers**

- **Sex helps to tighten women's pelvic-floor muscles, which improves bladder control**

- **Regular sex reduces the risk of prostate cancer**

- **Sleep often comes more quickly after orgasm.**

Watch less TV

Most adults watch TV for more than 2 hours a day. Spending too much time sitting down is bad for the heart, even for those of us who take regular exercise, so it shouldn't be too much of a surprise that a study found that every hour spent watching television increases your risk of dying.

People in the study who watched TV for 5 hours or more each day were 2.5 times more likely to die during the study period from a pulmonary embolism (a blood clot in the lung) compared with people who watched TV for fewer than 2.5 hours a day.

However, a recent meta-analysis has come up with a positive finding. If you limit your TV viewing to a maximum of 2 hours a day, from birth, you would live on average 1.4 years longer than people do now.

So, for a healthier and longer life, watch fewer box sets!

Change bed sheets regularly

Although there's very little scientific data on this matter, there is a good level of agreement about why changing bed linen is important. In fact, after washing your hands and your food, laundry hygiene is probably the next most important.

Each of us sheds millions of skin cells every day, many of them in bed. Typically, we shed 10 g of skin a day. In addition we produce 100 litres of sweat every year, which seeps into our bedding. This moisture is an ideal culture medium for fungi. Skin cells and sweat on sheets also attract dust mites, and dust mite droppings contain allergens that can trigger asthma, a runny nose and itchy eyes. Other nasties in your sheets include body oil, bacteria, soil, sputum (saliva and mucus coughed up from the respiratory tract), vaginal juice and even urine or worse.

A consensus is that changing your bed sheets once a week and washing them at a high temperature is ideal.

Develop good sleep hygiene

Good sleep hygiene – that's just another way of saying a **good pre-bedtime routine** – is important for a good night's sleep. Useful tips to achieve this:

- **Go to bed at the same time each day**
- **Get up at the same time each day**
- **Take regular exercise each day, but not late in the evening**
- **Keep the temperature comfortable in the bedroom**
- **Keep the bedroom dark**

- Keep the bedroom quiet

- Use the bedroom only for sleep, sex and reading, never for TV

- Do a relaxation exercise, e.g. meditation or yoga, just before going to sleep. Mindfulness is excellent

- Have a warm bath before bed

- Avoid stimulating activity just before bed, e.g. computer games, exciting TV programmes or movies, or important discussions

- Avoid watching tablets during the hour before bed

- Avoid caffeine (coffee, tea, chocolate and cola) in the evening

- Avoid (too much) alcohol in the evening. It may make you feel drowsy but its metabolites are a stimulant and are likely to wake you

- **Avoid going to bed either too hungry or too full**

- **Avoid trying to make yourself go to sleep as this will only make your mind more alert**

- **If you lie awake in bed for more than 20–30 minutes, get up and do something that isn't stimulating, e.g. reading a dull book, then go back to bed when you feel sleepy.**

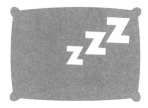

Have sufficient sleep

How much sleep adults need is one of the most debated health issues.

The National Sleep Foundation's recommended sleep ranges are:

- **Teenagers (14–17): 8–10 hours**
- **Adults (18–64): 7–9 hours**
- **Older adults (65+): 7–8 hours.**

Ask yourself:

- **How productive, healthy and happy am I on the amount of sleep I'm currently getting?**

- **Am I overweight?**

- **Am I experiencing sleep problems?**

- **Do I need caffeine to get through the day?**

- **Do I feel sleepy when driving?**

If the answer to most of these questions is yes, **consulting your doctor** is the next step to find a solution.

If you're experiencing symptoms such as sleepiness during the day, or if you snore or find yourself gasping or having difficulty breathing during sleep, see the next entry.

Snoring may be a red flag

Snoring is often the subject of jokes, yet not only is it not very funny but it can signal a serious health problem. Snoring is very closely related to **obstructive sleep apnoea** (OSA), when the throat narrows or closes during sleep and repeatedly interrupts your breathing – a condition that can increase the risks of high blood pressure, coronary heart disease, stroke and diabetes.

This simple questionnaire can help diagnose OSA. Use the following scale to choose the most appropriate number for how likely you are to doze off or fall asleep in each situation as opposed to just feeling tired. Answer each question as best you can.

Scale
0 = I would never doze
1 = slight chance of dozing
2 = moderate chance of dozing
3 = high chance of dozing

Situation	Chance of dozing
Sitting and reading	0 1 2 3
Watching TV	0 1 2 3
Sitting still in a public place (e.g. a theatre, a cinema or in a meeting)	0 1 2 3
Being a passenger in a car for an hour without a break	0 1 2 3
Lying down to rest in the afternoon when the circumstances allow	0 1 2 3

Sitting and talking to someone	0 1 2 3
Sitting quietly after lunch without having drunk alcohol	0 1 2 3
Being in a stationary car or bus for a few minutes in traffic	0 1 2 3
TOTAL	

A score of **16 or more** indicates that you're subject to **significant daytime sleepiness**. This could be due to obstructive sleep apnoea or another underlying medical condition that should be investigated. Please **consult your doctor**.

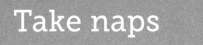

Take naps

Naps can be beneficial, although they can also have drawbacks. Look at these benefits and risks and if you think napping is for you, give it a try following the advice below.

Cautionary note
If you're experiencing an increased need for naps and there's no obvious cause in your life of new fatigue, consult your doctor.

The benefits of naps (according to a lot of evidence) include:

- **Less fatigue**
- **Relaxation**
- **Increased alertness**
- **Improved mood**
- **Improved performance and memory.**

The drawbacks of naps include:

- **Sleep inertia – feeling groggy and disorientated after waking up from a nap**
- **Night-time sleep problems. Short naps don't affect most people, but long or frequent naps can interfere with sleeping at night.**

The best way to take a nap

- Nap for no more than 30 minutes, ideally mid-afternoon when you're most likely to feel daytime sleepiness or a lower level of alertness

- After napping, make sure you have sufficient time to wake up before resuming your activities.

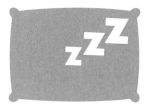

Don't smoke

Around **100,000 people** in the UK die each year from smoking.

Many more suffer from debilitating smoking-related diseases and issues including:

- **Damage to the heart and arteries, resulting in coronary heart disease, heart attack, stroke, poor circulation in the limbs and brain**
- **Damage to the lungs, resulting in chronic bronchitis and emphysema**
- **Many forms of cancer, including of the lung, mouth, oesophagus, larynx, stomach and bladder**

- **The risks associated with smoking before and during pregnancy, including miscarriage, low birth weight, premature babies and stillbirth.**

There are three stages to giving up smoking:

1. **Preparing to quit**

- **Smoking is strongly linked to certain situations, e.g. coffee breaks and phone calls. Break the link between these events and your smoking**

- **Decide on a day to stop. The day before, get rid of all your cigarettes and ashtrays**

- **Plan a reward for the end of your first day, first week and first month of being cigarette-free**

- Discuss with your GP quitting aids such as nicotine chewing gum and nicotine patches
- Join a local self-help group for support.

2. Quitting
- Take it one day at a time – your goal is to get through the day without smoking. Don't worry about tomorrow
- Congratulate yourself on having made it so far.

3. Staying smoke-free
- Think positive
- Remember why you decided to quit
- Ask your friends and family to keep encouraging you
- Reward yourself
- Don't be tempted to have the occasional cigarette – this would only reawaken the craving.

Have a regular blood test

A blood test can tell you a lot about your state of health. Regardless of how you feel physically, a comprehensive test is a good idea – **every two years** if you're under the age of 50, then **annually**.

I suggest you ask your doctor to test at least the following:

- **Haemoglobin (the pigment in red blood cells; see p.113)**
- **Red and white blood cells and clotting factors**
- **Kidney function**
- **Liver function**
- **Thyroid function**

- **Uric acid (to check for increased risk of gout)**
- **HbA1c (the test for diabetes)**
- **Blood lipids (cholesterol and triglycerides)**
- **Vitamin B12, folate and vitamin D**
- **For men over 50, PSA (prostate-specific antigen).**

If the test highlights any problem areas, your GP will be able to help you address them.

Have a regular urine test

The purpose of the urine test is to indicate the presence of the following, none of which should normally be present:

- **Blood**
- **Glucose (sugar)**
- **Protein.**

Blood or protein in urine can be a sign of **infection** or may indicate kidney or bladder disease.

The presence of glucose (sugar) in the urine may be the first sign of **diabetes**. Because diabetes can go undiagnosed for ten years or more, it's a good idea to ask your doctor to check your urine **annually** – a simple dipstick test that takes less than a minute.

Know your cholesterol level

The **higher** your cholesterol, the **greater** the risk of coronary heart disease and stroke, so knowing your numbers is really important.

And it's not just your total cholesterol – that's the one that should be less than 5 mmol/L (the unit of measurement for blood lipids) – that matters. It's quite possible to have a total cholesterol level that is much higher – 6 or even 7 mmol/L – without any increased risk.

To get a true picture, you need to drill down to the different types of cholesterol. LDL is the 'bad' cholesterol that clogs up arteries. Ideally this should be 3 mmol/L or less. HDL is the protective cholesterol – the more you have of this, the better. This should be at least 1.2 mmol/L.

But the most important number is the percentage of HDL. This should be at least 25 per cent of total cholesterol, preferably 33 per cent or more.

As an example, let's take Frank. He's 53 years old and has a total cholesterol level of 5.6, which seems a little high. His LDL is 3.5 – also a little high. But his HDL is 2.5 – this is really high and excellent. HDL forms 45 per cent of his total cholesterol, so overall his cholesterol is fine.

To lower LDL, eat less saturated fat – red meat, butter, whole milk and cheese, etc. To increase HDL, eat less saturated fat (as above), take more exercise and don't smoke.

Get tested for type 2 diabetes

Insulin resistance is when your body stops using insulin properly. Insulin is made in the pancreas but eventually the pancreas is no longer able to produce enough insulin, and this condition is type 2 diabetes.

Insulin keeps your blood glucose (blood sugar) at normal levels. If blood glucose levels become too high, which is what happens in diabetes, several health problems result. In particular, there can be damage to the eyes, heart, kidneys and nerves.

Unfortunately, because there are typically no symptoms of the disease for long periods, type 2 diabetes often goes undiagnosed for 10–15 years, by which time a lot of damage has already been done. This is why it's important to **ask your doctor** to test you for diabetes and prediabetes, particularly if you're at high risk – if you have a

family history of type 2 diabetes, if you're **significantly overweight** or from an **Asian background**.

There are several ways of checking for diabetes. A simple, initial screening tests whether there's glucose in the urine. A better test is to measure the level of glucose in the blood while fasting. But the gold standard is to measure the HbA1c. This is a form of haemoglobin that tells us the average blood glucose concentration in the previous two to three months.

Lifestyle changes, such as adopting a low-GI diet and taking more exercise, may slow down the progression to type 2 diabetes or even prevent it altogether, so early diagnosis of diabetes – or, even better, of prediabetes – is one of the most important steps for maintaining a long and healthy life.

URBAN MYTH:
Artificial sweeteners make you fat

This is another common myth, especially since a research paper (published in 2015) attracted media attention. The paper, published in the *Journal of the American Geriatric Society*, concluded that diet soda, which contains artificial sweeteners, is associated with increasing abdominal girth.

But consider this: the study was done on over-65s, many of whom were already overweight and quite a few were type 2 diabetics who were anxious to avoid sugar.

Experts at Addenbrooke's Hospital and St George's Hospital are **very sceptical** of the paper's conclusions, as am I.

Know your haemoglobin

There are many reasons why your haemoglobin level may be low. A high haemoglobin level is less common.

Possible reasons for a low haemoglobin level:

- **You're producing fewer red blood cells than usual. Possible causes include vitamin deficiency (especially folate, vitamin B-12 or vitamin C), iron deficiency, cystitis, aplastic anaemia, Hodgkin's disease, myeloma, an underactive thyroid, cirrhosis, chronic kidney disease and various forms of cancer**

- You're destroying red blood cells faster than normal because you have e.g. a urinary tract infection, an enlarged spleen or thalassaemia

- You're losing blood, due to e.g. heavy periods, bleeding from the bowel because of haemorrhoids or cancer.

Possible reasons for a high haemoglobin level:

- Smoking
- Chronic lung disease
- Kidney cancer
- Liver cancer
- Heart failure

- **Polycythaemia vera (a type of blood cancer in which the bone marrow makes too many red blood cells).**

Because there are so many causes of an abnormal haemoglobin, and because some of them are not only quite common but also serious (such as bowel cancer), it's a good idea to have a **regular blood test** – say, every two years until the age of 50 and then annually. Ask your doctor to do other tests on your blood at the same time (see p.105).

Check your blood pressure once a year

Most strokes are preventable. Because **high blood pressure** is the main cause of strokes, it's important to make sure yours is normal in order to give yourself the greatest chance possible of preventing a stroke.

Guidelines say that 140/90 or less is a normal blood pressure, but 120/80 or less is ideal.

But what do these figures mean? The higher figure is called 'systolic blood pressure'. This is the pressure in your arteries as blood is pumped out of the heart – you feel this as a heartbeat. The lower figure is the 'diastolic blood pressure'. This is the pressure in your arteries when the heart relaxes between heartbeats.

Ideally you should keep both figures **as low as possible**, something that is largely down to a healthy lifestyle – not being overweight, not drinking too much alcohol, taking plenty of exercise and avoiding adding more than just a small amount of salt to food.

Despite a healthy lifestyle, many people develop high blood pressure, especially as they grow older. Doctors then prescribe **medication** to lower blood pressure. If blood pressure is high enough to need medication, it's vital to take the prescribed drugs and never to stop them unless advised to do so by a doctor (which rarely happens).

You absolutely cannot monitor your blood pressure by how you feel. The *only* way to know if blood pressure is high or not is by measuring it with a blood pressure machine.

It scares me how many people are so casual about their blood pressure. It's very important to ask your doctor to measure blood pressure regularly (an **annual 'MOT'** is a good idea) and, if necessary, to take prescribed medication daily.

Check your heart

Although a full physical examination and tests are the only way to thoroughly check the state of your heart, this option isn't practical or affordable for many of us.

The good news is that there are some good online tools. The excellent online calculator and downloadable app (for iOS and Android) QRISK®2 gives you a good idea of which aspects of your lifestyle you can change for the good of your heart. To use it, you will need to know your height (in metres), weight (in kilograms), total cholesterol, HDL ('good') cholesterol and blood pressure.

QRISK®2 will quantify your ten-year risk of developing coronary heart disease or stroke. If the result is higher than typical for your age, sex and ethnicity – and the tool will tell you this – then it would be a good idea to discuss this with your doctor.

Take a low dose of aspirin daily – perhaps

The number-one condition that people have in mind when thinking about taking 75 mg aspirin daily (low dose aspirin) is **CVS disease** (cardiovascular disease), i.e. coronary heart disease and stroke.

When doctors consider the prevention of CVS disease, they think about two different situations:

- **Primary prevention – preventing disease in those who have never had a problem**

- **Secondary prevention – preventing further disease in those who already have CVS disease, i.e. those who've suffered a heart attack, angina or stroke.**

NICE, the UK government health quango whose guidelines doctors tend to follow, says that low dose aspirin should be used for secondary prevention, but not for primary prevention. This is because the risks of low dose aspirin (mainly bleeding from the gut), though small, outweigh the benefits in those with CVS disease.

Other people who might benefit from low dose aspirin:

- **Women who are over 12 weeks pregnant and taking long-haul flights. This is controversial and should be done only on the advice of a doctor**

- **Pregnant women with a history of pre-eclampsia or high blood pressure in pregnancy – again, only on a doctor's advice**

- **Women with a history of three or more unexplained miscarriages.**

A very important note

If you think you would benefit from low dose aspirin, always check with your doctor first as aspirin can have serious side effects (bleeding and allergic reactions). Aspirin should never be given to children under the age of 16.

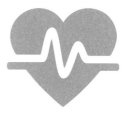

Guys, check your testicles

It constantly amazes me how few men check their testicles. Patients ask me about having this test and that test for cancer, but something as simple as checking their testicles seems to escape so many.

The best time to self-examine is during or just after a bath or shower, when the skin of the scrotum is relaxed. One at a time, hold each testicle between the thumbs and first two fingers of both hands. Roll each testicle gently between the fingers. Look for any lumps that have appeared since the last self-exam or any changes in the size, shape or consistency of each testicle.

Doing a regular self-exam once a month means you become familiar with how the testicles should feel and enables you to recognise any changes early on.

The worst possible cause of a change is **testicular cancer**, which affects mainly, but not exclusively, men aged 20–40. Non-cancer changes may be due to infection, a cyst, a varicocele (an enlargement of the veins within the scrotum), a hydrocele (a fluid-filled sac surrounding a testicle that results in swelling in the scrotum) or even a hernia. However, **don't try to make a diagnosis yourself** – any change should always be checked by a **doctor**, who may recommend a scan.

If the change is testicular cancer, the chances of complete cure are greatest if the tumour is **diagnosed and treated early**.

Guys, get your prostate checked – or should you?

Prostate cancer is the top health concern that I hear about from most middle-aged men, and prostate-cancer testing is the most common cancer-screening request that doctors get from men.

Some doctors advocate testing by feeling the prostate through the rectum, but the value of this is controversial. What is undoubtedly more useful is the **PSA (prostate-specific antigen) blood test**. An antigen is a molecule that induces an immune response – if there is prostate cancer, a man's immune system produces more antibodies.

PSA testing is also controversial, and this is for several reasons. A raised PSA may be due to non-cancer causes, such as infection or an energetic bout of sexual activity in the preceding 48 hours. Prostate cancer may be present despite a normal PSA, although this is very rare. And even if a raised PSA is due to the presence of cancer, the vast majority of men with prostate cancer don't die of the disease – they die *with* the cancer, not *because of* the cancer.

A raised PSA level often requires further investigations, such as an **MRI scan** and **prostate biopsy**. Although these may be uncomfortable procedures, they are worthwhile as they can help diagnose and lead to early treatment for cancer.

Personally, I believe that all men should be tested **from age 50 onwards**, though not all doctors will agree. Certainly any man with a **family history of prostate cancer** (if his father, grandfather, uncle or brother has had prostate cancer), or any man with **urinary symptoms**, such as a burning sensation during urination or blood in the urine, should consider being tested.

Ladies, don't miss your cervical smear tests

Although cancer is one of the main health concerns today, the sad fact is that there are very few cancers that can be screened for. In women, breast and cervical cancer are the two most important.

Routine cervical cancer screening is available to all women from age 25. It's a simple procedure that's generally painless, although it may be uncomfortable.

A doctor or nurse passes a plastic speculum into the vagina. A small brush is inserted to sweep the cervix (the neck of the womb) for cells. The specimen is sent to a laboratory where it's checked for suspicious cells. The lab also checks for the presence of HPV (human papillomavirus), which can cause cervical cancer.

If abnormal cells are found, or if HPV is present, the smear test is likely to be repeated in three to six months, although in certain cases another procedure, **colposcopy**, may be advised. Colposcopy is a safe procedure which takes no more than 5–10 minutes and doesn't require an anaesthetic.

Under the NHS, cervical smears are carried out every three years, but some women feel happier having the test more often, which can be done in private practice.

Cervical cancer screening is crucial. If abnormal cells are detected early, a potentially life-threatening illness can be prevented or cured.

Ladies, check your breasts regularly

Breast cancer is the **most common cancer** in the UK.

While some experts disagree about the importance of regular breast self-examination, most doctors agree that it's a good idea to get into the habit of checking your breasts **once a month**, preferably at the end of each period. There are lots of good videos on YouTube which demonstrate the best way to do this.

In simple terms, stand in front of a mirror. Look at your breasts with your arms at your sides. Next, raise your arms over your head. Look for any changes in the contour of each breast, or any swelling or dimpling of the skin, or changes in the nipples.

Next, lie down. A bath is a good place to do this. Using the pads of your three middle fingers, move around your entire breast in a spiral pattern, working from the outside to the centre, checking the entire breast and armpit area. Feel for lumps or thickening, or an area of deep tenderness. Gently squeeze the nipple to make sure there's no blood or discharge. Repeat for the other breast.

If you think you can feel a lump, *don't panic* – **most lumps are benign**, usually cysts or lumps of fibrous tissue – but always seek medical advice.

The NHS invites women to have a **mammogram** as a breast-cancer-screening test **every three years from age 50**. However, if you have an immediate family history of breast cancer, you should consider having a mammogram **every 18 months from age 40** – you may have to arrange this privately.

These days, the outlook for most cases of breast cancer is excellent if the condition is diagnosed early.

Get checked for bowel cancer

Bowel cancer is the fourth most common cancer in the UK – after breast, prostate and lung cancer. Over 40,000 people are diagnosed with bowel cancer every year in the UK. Most cases are in people over the age of 50.

The NHS offers bowel-cancer screening **every two years** to all adults aged 60 or over. If you're prepared to pay, screening is available at any age.

A simple test can detect the presence of occult blood (hidden blood resulting from cancer or precancerous lesions in the bowel) in the stools, which can then be further investigated to rule out cancer. A home-testing kit is used to collect tiny stool samples on a special card. The card is then sent to the laboratory in a special envelope. The samples are checked for traces of blood that could be an early sign of bowel cancer.

Blood in the stools can be a sign of any condition that causes bleeding into the digestive tract (e.g. an ulcer, polyps or diverticulitis). The result will either be negative (no blood) or positive (blood found).

In **98 per cent** of people, blood in the stools suggests an easily treated condition. In only **2 per cent** of people with a positive test, blood in the stools is a sign of bowel cancer.

Check for moles

Learn the ABCDEs of **melanoma**. A melanoma is cancer that develops from melanocytes, which are pigment-containing cells.

Look for these signs in new or existing moles:

- **Asymmetry:** melanoma lesions are often irregular, or not symmetrical, in shape. Benign moles are usually symmetrical

- **Border:** typically, non-cancerous moles have smooth, even borders. Melanoma lesions usually have irregular borders that are difficult to define

- **Colour:** the presence of more than one colour (blue, black, brown or tan, etc.) or the uneven distribution of colour can sometimes be a warning sign of melanoma. Benign moles are usually a single shade of brown or tan

- **Diameter:** melanoma lesions are often greater than 6 mm in diameter (approximately the size of a pencil-top eraser)

- **Evolution:** the evolution of your mole(s) has become the most important factor to consider when it comes to diagnosing a melanoma. Knowing what is normal for *you* could save your life. If a mole has gone through recent changes in colour and/or size, bring it to the attention of a dermatologist (skin specialist) immediately.

Promptly tell your doctor about **any changes** to a mole. If you have a lot of moles, ask your doctor to refer you to a dermatologist, who can carry out a detailed mole check using a dermatoscope, a special magnifier that allows more accurate inspection of skin lesions.

Use sunscreen

The risk of skin cancer increases with damage to the skin from **UVA** and **UVB** (the two types of ultraviolet radiation). UVB is the chief culprit behind sunburn, while UVA rays, which penetrate the skin more deeply, are associated with wrinkling and other sun-related ageing effects on the skin.

SPF is a measure of how well a sunscreen prevents UVB from damaging the skin, e.g. an SPF 30 sunscreen theoretically protects the skin for 30 times longer than it would usually take for your skin to burn. So, say it takes 20 minutes for your unprotected skin to start turning red, then using an SPF 30 sunscreen theoretically prevents reddening for about 10 hours.

Sunscreens vary in their ability to protect against UVA and UVB. Most sunscreens with an SPF of 15 or higher are good at protecting against

UVB. Broad-spectrum sunscreens protect the skin from both UVA and UVB rays – always check the label.

> Use a 'high protection' sunscreen of at least SPF 30 which also has high UVA protection. Ensure that you apply it generously and often when in the sun, following the guidelines on the packaging.

While a sunscreen is very important, even more important are a few simple measures for sunny days:

- **Stay in the shade between 11 a.m. and 3 p.m.**

- **Wear long clothes and a hat to protect your head and skin**

- **Wear sunglasses – your eyes also need protection from UV radiation.**

Check for osteoporosis

One in two women and **one in five men** over the age of 50 will break a bone as a result of osteoporosis.

Osteoporosis is a condition in which the bones become brittle and fragile as a result of loss of tissue. This is usually because of hormonal changes or deficiency of calcium and/or vitamin D.

If you have osteoporosis, broken bones are more likely to occur after even a simple fall. The most common bones to be affected are the wrist, the hip and the spine. One particular concern about a hip fracture in an elderly person is that it can result in them becoming more frail, which can reduce life expectancy.

A great way to see if you're at risk of osteoporosis is to use the **QFracture**® online risk calculator at **qfracture.org** (you will need to know your height and weight). It's a good idea to use this tool every three years from the age of 30.

Ways to reduce the risk of osteoporosis:

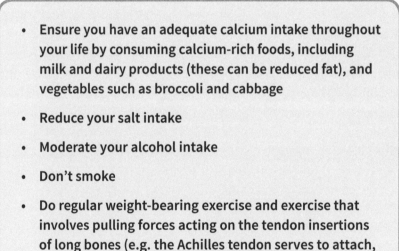

- **Ensure you have an adequate calcium intake throughout your life by consuming calcium-rich foods, including milk and dairy products (these can be reduced fat), and vegetables such as broccoli and cabbage**

- **Reduce your salt intake**

- **Moderate your alcohol intake**

- **Don't smoke**

- **Do regular weight-bearing exercise and exercise that involves pulling forces acting on the tendon insertions of long bones (e.g. the Achilles tendon serves to attach, or insert, the calf muscles to the heel).**

Have a regular eye check

Visiting the optician isn't just about getting a pair of prescription glasses – in fact, that's its least important value when looking at your overall health. An optometrist (the professional who looks at your eyes and tests your vision) can check whether there are both any problems with your eyes and with your general health.

There are several eye problems which you won't necessarily be aware of until you have an eye test. One is **glaucoma**, which is raised pressure in the eye. Untreated, it can lead to blindness. Incidentally, anyone whose parents have glaucoma is entitled to free eye checks in the UK. Sight tests can also check for an eye condition called **macular degeneration** (an important cause of visual loss), and **cataracts**, which these days are very quick and simple to treat – a day-case surgical procedure, often under local anaesthetic.

An eye test may also reveal changes in the retina, especially the blood vessels, and the presence of tiny haemorrhages which can indicate general health problems – notable examples are diabetes and high blood pressure.

Ideally, you should have an eye test **every two years**. However, those over 70, or those over 40 with a family history of glaucoma should have an **annual test**.

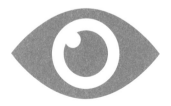

Regularly brush and floss your teeth

Dentists advise brushing teeth for **two minutes twice a day** (results are best with an electric toothbrush), and flossing or using an interdental brush or toothpick between your teeth **once a day**. But brushing and flossing aren't just about caring for your teeth.

Numerous health problems can arise from poor oral hygiene:

- **Dental disease – this can take a variety of forms, including gum disease and plaque. If plaque spreads, the immune response heightens and can destroy tissues and bones in the mouth. Poor oral hygiene can cause cavities and gum disease, which can result in tooth loss. And although** other conditions may cause bad breath (halitosis), poor oral hygiene is by far the most common cause

- Ulcers and cancer – research points to poor oral hygiene leading to the growth of *Helicobacter pylori* bacteria, which can result in stomach ulcers and cancer of the mouth and stomach

- Heart disease – certainly there is a link between gum disease and heart disease, but whether the gum disease leads to heart disease or whether there is simply a common cause for both remains a controversial topic

- Kidney disease – this is four to five times more common in those with dental disease

- Brain abscess – poor oral hygiene can lead to an abscess anywhere in the body. A brain abscess can be fatal

- Diabetes – diabetes may be a risk factor for dental disease and recent research suggests that dental disease may be a risk factor for prediabetes (insulin resistance)

- **Pneumonia** – research points to an increased risk of pneumonia in those with poor oral hygiene

- **Dementia** – research suggests there is a possible link between poor dental health and dementia. One study found that the brains of Alzheimer's patients contained more bacteria associated with gum disease than those without Alzheimer's

- **Pregnancy complications** – there's a link between dental disease and low birth weight and preterm birth

- **Erectile dysfunction** – this may seem an odd association, but research suggests there could be a link.

Eating more than three eggs a week is bad for you

Eggs are a good source of protein, vitamins and minerals. They're also rich in betaine and choline, which promote heart health. Yet eggs have had a bad press for decades.

We have variously been told:

- **In the 1970s: go to work on an egg**

- **In the 1980s: there is salmonella in most eggs**

- **In the 1990s: eating eggs raises your cholesterol.**

Eggs are high in cholesterol, but the cholesterol they contain is not as harmful as the saturated fat from meat – and it is the saturated fat, not cholesterol, in your diet that increases the level of cholesterol in your blood. Your liver makes many times more cholesterol than you get from eating eggs. Eggs contain some saturated fat, but the butter on your toast or the bacon that may accompany your eggs have a far greater impact on cholesterol.

So are there any benefits to eating only the whites, as in egg-white omelettes?

- **No – if your concern is cholesterol**
- **Yes – if your concern is controlling your weight, since egg yolks are very calorific.**

Eating eggs during pregnancy

At one time the risk of salmonella (a bacterium that causes food poisoning) in eggs was quite significant, so the advice used to be to avoid eating raw or lightly cooked eggs during pregnancy. However, recently the Advisory Committee on the Microbiological Safety of Food has said that the risk of salmonella from UK eggs produced to the Lion Code (or equivalent) standards should be considered 'very low'. Nevertheless, to be absolutely safe, it is still probably wise to cook eggs until the whites and yolks are solid.

Stay out of hospital

Hospitals can be dangerous places, especially for the elderly. Five thousand people die every year due to infections picked up in UK hospitals.

The most common hospital-acquired infections include:

- **Bloodstream infections, complicating IV treatment (intravenous infusions)**
- **Urinary tract infections in catheterised patients**
- **Surgical-site infections after surgery**

- **Superbug infections:**
  - *Clostridium difficile* (*C. diff*): these bacteria live in the bowel without causing symptoms, but if the immune system is weakened they can cause significant infections that are becoming increasingly resistant to antibiotics

  - Methicillin-resistant and Vancomycin-resistant *Staphylococcus aureus* (MRSA and VRSA): these bacteria can lead to sepsis (a severe, potentially life-threatening condition with symptoms typically including fever, increased heart rate and increased breathing rate) and death.

Hospitals are essential places, where lives are saved and serious medical conditions are treated – but if you don't need to be there, try to avoid them.

Exercise your brain

Research shows that mental activity can reduce your risk of dementia. Any activity that involves thinking and learning may be beneficial for brain health.

Studies show that greater benefit comes from more complex and challenging mental activities. The more brain activities you do, the more often you do them and the more complex the activity, the lower your risk of dementia is likely to be.

It's best to choose activities that challenge your brain and give you enjoyment as well – boring activities aren't healthy for your brain.

Examples of good mental activities:

- Reading a variety of books, newspapers and magazines

- Doing crosswords and number or word puzzles

- Playing cards or board games

- Going to the theatre, movies, concerts, museums and galleries

- Researching something interesting on the internet

- Cooking a new recipe

- Learning a new language

- Learning to play a musical instrument

- Taking up a new hobby, such as painting, carpentry, metalwork or sewing

- Joining a club or community group or volunteering.

Develop a positive attitude

Research has demonstrated that cultivating **positivity** can not only lengthen your life but also improve the **quality** of your life.

Benefits of a positive attitude include:

- **Happiness**
- **Greater self-motivation**
- **More energy**
- **Better health**
- **Improved productivity**
- **Ability to handle stress more easily**

- **Stronger relationships**
- **Respect from other people.**

Ways to develop a positive attitude:

- **Be happy – don't wait for something to happen to make you happy. Happiness is an attitude, not a situation**

- **Enjoy the small pleasures of life – e.g. watching the sunset and supper in your favourite restaurant**

- **Focus on the good in your life – be grateful that you're alive, that you have a family, friends and a job, etc.**

- **Smile – smiling immediately boosts your attitude because it releases endorphins and serotonin ('happy hormones'), which make it easier to be positive.**

Try smiling for a few moments while you recall a happy memory

- Upload positive thoughts to your brain – read a book that carries an upbeat message, watch a film in which the protagonist wins despite the odds, or listen to a song with uplifting lyrics

- Take responsibility for your life instead of being a victim – tell yourself that you're responsible for yourself and in charge of your own destiny

- Have purpose and meaning in your life

- Don't expect life to be easy – rather see life as a series of challenges that will make you a stronger person

- Visualise yourself as the happy, successful person you want to be

- Surround yourself with people who have a positive outlook – positivity is infectious.

Make yourself happy

Happiness has been the subject of considerable medical research – academic institutions that have published reports on this subject include Harvard University and the University of California, Berkeley. Researchers think of happiness as having **satisfaction** and **meaning** in your life.

Use the mnemonic **GATES** to help you remember how to be happy:

GIVE. In one study, students were asked to perform five random acts of kindness each week for six weeks, and these people felt more than a 40 per cent increase in happiness. Being kind makes you feel less stressed, isolated and angry as well as much happier

ASPIRE. Research shows that people who create meaning in their lives are happier. Feeling hopeful and optimistic and having a sense of purpose lead to greater satisfaction

THANK. Studies show that people who write thank-you letters to someone they've never properly thanked before immediately feel much happier and have fewer symptoms of depression

EMPATHISE. Compassion is a skill that can be learned. Caring about others makes you less judgemental and disappointed in how others behave towards and around you. Empathy strengthens your bonds – and strong relationships are vital for happiness. People who show more compassion lead healthier and more productive lives

SAVOUR. Research has shown that the practice of being mindful and noticing the good stuff around you, taking the extra time to intensify your enjoyment of the moment, boosts optimism and reduces stress and negative emotions. You can savour the past (by reminiscing), savour the future (through positive anticipation) or savour the present (by practising mindfulness).

Follow the happiness diet

Research shows that there is a link between **diet** and **mood**. Eating certain foods may protect your brain from depression.

Here are some ways to follow the happiness diet:

- **Fuel your brain with glucose, which is so important for regulating mood. Choose slow-releasing or wholegrain carbohydrates, e.g. oat porridge; legumes (beans, lentils and chickpeas); fruit and low-fat yoghurt**

- **Eat oily fish two to three times a week or take an omega-3 supplement. Research shows that people with** depression tend to have lower levels of omega-3 fats in their diet. Good fish sources include salmon, mackerel, sardines and tuna. Good non-fish sources include canola oil, linseed oil, soybean oil and walnuts

- Consume foods containing the amino acid tryptophan. Tryptophan is converted to serotonin, a 'happy hormone' and a brain chemical that improves mood. Good food sources include: red meat; milk; eggs; nuts; lentils; wholegrain bread, cereals and pasta; and dark chocolate (but only have a little chocolate because too much isn't healthy)

- Follow a Mediterranean-style diet – a diet rich in vegetables, fruit, wholegrains, nuts, fish, olive oil and low-fat unsweetened yoghurt. This seems to be linked to lower rates of depression compared with diets which contain a lot of processed foods

- Try these dietary mood-enhancing ideas:

  ○ Eat a small tub of low-fat yoghurt with a piece of fruit

- Add a boiled egg to a salad

- Combine a tin of tuna or salmon or sardines with sliced tomato on crunchy multigrain crackers

- Snack on a few walnuts with two fresh dates

- Crunch on some raw vegetable sticks with hummus.

Laugh a lot

'Laughter is the best medicine' is an old saying, but how true is it? When you laugh, your pulse quickens and you breathe faster, which sends more **oxygen** to your tissues – which is important to help provide **energy** and for survival.

Some fitness experts reckon that **1 minute** of laughter increases the heart rate to the same extent that **10 minutes** on a rowing machine does, and research shows that 10–15 minutes of laughter burns around **50 calories**.

Other benefits of laughter include:

- Better blood flow, which may help protect against heart disease

- A boosted immune system

- The release of endorphins, which leads to better relaxation and sleep

- Can aid pain relief

- Lowered blood sugar levels

- Laughing with others helps bonding and teamwork, leading to a happier and less stressful work environment.

Embrace life's challenges

Life is full of ups and downs, highs and lows. It's important not to let the lows destroy your sense of joy and govern your feelings, and it's a good idea to learn to handle these challenges with a minimal amount of stress.

Think of challenging circumstances as a way of teaching you to adopt a **positive mindset** and practise **mindfulness**. If you practise trying to enjoy every moment of every day whatever life throws at you, you can become better at enjoying the here and now.

Focus on **solutions** rather than problems. This helps promote happiness, which boosts your immune system, protecting you from illness and giving you a **longer life**.

Do some good

The **golden rule** or the **law of reciprocity** is the principle of treating others as one would wish to be treated oneself. We've all heard that it's better to give than receive, but here's an interesting fact: this is backed up by research.

The evidence shows that helping others is also beneficial for your own mental health and well-being – it can reduce stress and even boost your physical health.

The health benefits of helping others:

- **Promotes positive physiological changes in the brain that are associated with happiness**

- **Leads to a sense of belonging. Volunteering that involves face-to-face activities can reduce feelings of loneliness and isolation**

- **Can make you realise how lucky you are, especially if you help those who are less fortunate than yourself**

- **Can last a long time, by providing a 'kindness bank' of memories that you can draw upon**

- **Helps you mentally because positive emotions reduce stress and boost your immune system, in turn protecting you against disease**

- **May increase your life expectancy. Research shows that those who support others live longer.**

Several ways you can do good

- Volunteering

- Mentoring and counselling

- Being involved with a good cause

- Doing random acts of kindness at home and at work.

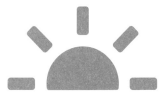

Have a sense of higher purpose

In Viktor Frankl's book *Man's Search for Meaning*, the author describes his experiences in concentration camps during the Second World War. He observed that the prisoners who were most likely to survive were those who had a **goal** or **purpose**.

The need for purpose is one of the defining characteristics of human beings. Without purpose, you may become more vulnerable to boredom, anxiety and depression. This can lead to physical and mental health problems and a shortened life.

Research shows that people with a high sense of purpose have a lower risk of heart disease and stroke. With a sense of purpose, life becomes easier, less complicated and less stressful.

In another study, 9,000 people over the age of 65 were followed for 8.5 years. Researchers measured their well-being by giving them a questionnaire that gauged how much control they felt they had over their own life, and how much they thought what they did was worthwhile. The results showed that more contented people tended to outlive those who were less fulfilled. Over the 8.5 years, only 9 per cent of people in the highest well-being category died, compared to 29 per cent in the lowest category. These findings support previous research that has linked happiness to a longer life.

To find a sense of purpose, you need to understand what you love to do, what you feel passionate and curious about, plus what you feel is important.

These simple questions can help you define your purpose:

- **Who am I?**
- **What can I contribute to others?**

- If I had only a year left to live, how would I live my life?

- What are my beliefs and values?

- Over the past week, what have I done that has fully engaged me?

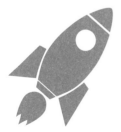

Don't retire early

Many of us might dream of a retirement spent travelling and trying out new hobbies, yet escaping the office in reality may make you more miserable and prone to sickness.

In 2013, France's federal health agency, INSERM, studied dementia prevalence among 429,000 people over the age of 60. Their findings? Jumping ship at 60 increased your risk of the illness by about 15 per cent, compared with those who waited an extra five years before hanging up their hats. They concluded that **work** keeps your brain **young** and **fit**, while early retirement is bad for your physical and emotional health.

Researchers from the London-based Institute of Economic Affairs think tank surveyed 9,000 adults aged 50–70 from 11 European countries. They found that on retirement the average adult is 60 per cent more likely to have at least one diagnosed illness than those still at work. Retirement also increases the risk of depression by 40 per cent and the chance of being on medication by 60 per cent. Retirees are 40 per cent less likely to declare themselves in either 'very good' or 'excellent' health than those still working.

The message for most of us is clear: don't retire too early.

Be a social butterfly

The pain of loneliness is a biological trigger, like hunger or pain. Hunger means you need to eat. Pain protects you from physical danger. According to neuroscientists and psychologists, loneliness is a warning that signals the need for change in order to restore something necessary for your genetic survival: it protects you from isolation.

One definition of loneliness is sadness because one has no friends or company. You can have many friends and social engagements yet still feel lonely. You can be married and feel lonely. It's the quality of your relationships, not the quantity, that counts.

Evidence suggests that isolation is more common than it was 20–30 years ago, with some studies suggesting that perhaps as many as 20 per cent of us feel unhappily isolated.

Loneliness is a problem for your health because, in general, lonely people tend to eat foods high in sugar and fat, and tend to have higher blood pressure and produce more stress hormones, all of which is damaging to health and can lead to premature death.

If you're lonely, you could try volunteering for charity work, joining social groups or engaging in activities to meet like-minded people and **make connections**. It may be easier said than done, but reaching out and trying your best to become a social butterfly will benefit your overall health.

Be married

Marriage (between people of any gender) has enormous benefits on health. Research shows that married people have a lower incidence of numerous health problems, including cancer and heart attacks, and a higher chance of recovery from major surgery such as heart bypass.

Married men have a 64 per cent lower chance of fatal strokes than single men, according to the American Stroke Association.

Married couples are less likely to engage in risky behaviour, such as substance abuse or dangerous driving, plus they're less likely to develop mental illness and they often sleep better.

A major study on almost 5,000 older individuals, conducted by researchers at Duke University Medical Centre, showed that having a partner through middle and old age is protective against premature

death. Those who never married were more than twice as likely to die early than those who had experienced a long, stable marriage throughout the majority of their adult life.

What about long-term relationships that don't involve marriage? The evidence certainly points to other significant relationships resulting in health benefits, but probably not to the same degree as marriage.

Finish off those annoying tasks

Have you been putting something off? Are you **procrastinating**? Is there a task that keeps niggling at the back of your mind? If so, it can leave you feeling unsettled, annoyed and stressed.

Going through life putting off annoying tasks creates a state of **tension**, which releases stress hormones – and a constant surge of stress hormones shortens lives by many years. The burden of leaving a lot of tasks unfinished can have the same cumulative impact on your health as a major life event, such as divorce or the death of a loved one.

Research shows that when you procrastinate, you might feel better in the short-term, but you will suffer in the **long-term**. Procrastination can cause depression, anxiety, stress and low self-esteem.

Finishing an irritating task lets you breathe a sigh of **relief**, makes you feel more at **peace** and may also turbocharge your energy levels.

Take more holidays

A survey published in 2011 showed that, on average, we need a holiday **six times a year** (or every 62 days) in order to avoid damaging levels of stress.

The survey showed that:

- **One in four of us admits to feeling stressed if we wait more than two months before taking a break**
- **One in five of us needs a holiday within a month of our last trip away**
- **Fifteen per cent of us admit that it takes at least five days to feel fully relaxed while on holiday**

- **Thirty per cent of us take just two week-long holidays throughout the year combined with regular long weekends**

- **Many of us need to take regular breaks in order to feel relaxed and recharged.**

Experts advise that we need **six weeks'** holiday a year to prevent **burnout**. Those who wait more than two months between holidays are more likely to become anxious, aggressive and ill. You're more likely to struggle to get to sleep, and you may also develop aches and pains. Overworking depresses your immune system, making it more likely that you will become ill. **So go ahead and book that holiday!**

Manage work stress

While it may not always feel like it, **working is healthy**. It keeps your brain active, improves your skills and provides you with social relationships.

But work can cause **stress**. Typical signs of stress are feeling demotivated or unable to cope, irritability, headaches, difficulty sleeping or chest pains.

Stress may be caused by being overworked, which is likely to be the situation if you work longer hours, take work home, spend less time with your family and friends or skip lunch.

Coping with stress puts you in control and enables you to live a **longer, happier life**.

Ways to cope with work stress:

- **Eat regular, balanced meals** – to keep blood sugar stable, as low blood sugar can make you feel irritable

- **Take regular exercise** – this releases endorphins (the 'happy hormones') which aid sleep and fight off depression

- **Spend more time with family and friends** – they're your support network and they'll notice if you show signs of stress

- **Avoid substances** – using nicotine and alcohol to improve your mood doesn't help in the long-term

- **Practise mindfulness** – this form of meditation helps you to focus on the present moment, which in turn helps you to avoid becoming stressed and can help you manage stress if it does happen. Mindfulness improves concentration and reduces feelings of stress and anxiety. There is an excellent mindfulness app called Headspace.

Practise more relaxation

While most of us need some stress to power us through the day, we also need **relaxation** to offset the damaging effects of stress hormones.

The benefits of relaxation include:

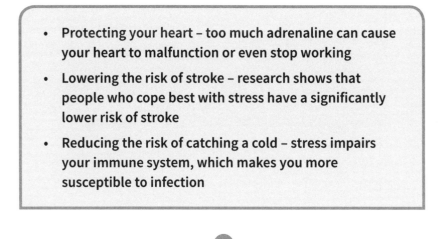

- **Protecting your heart – too much adrenaline can cause your heart to malfunction or even stop working**
- **Lowering the risk of stroke – research shows that people who cope best with stress have a significantly lower risk of stroke**
- **Reducing the risk of catching a cold – stress impairs your immune system, which makes you more susceptible to infection**

- **Lowering the likelihood of becoming overweight –** stress hormones increase your appetite and make it more difficult for you to resist comfort foods (foods that are high in fat and sugar)

- **Helping various skin conditions –** especially psoriasis and acne

- **Boosting memory –** research has shown that stress can impair the centres of the brain involved in memory and learning. There is also evidence that stress may accelerate the development of Alzheimer's

- **Lessening the risk of depression –** repeated exposure to stress hormones can reduce levels of serotonin and dopamine, which can result in depression

- **Helping you make better decisions –** when you're stressed you tend not to think so clearly. Stress can cloud your judgement when you're faced with important decisions.

There are many different ways to relax, and all take practice. Different techniques work for different people. Find one that works best for you.

Ways to relax

- Meditation or mindfulness
- Yoga
- Self-hypnosis
- Autogenic training (a desensitisation-relaxation technique)
- Read a book
- Take a bath
- Go for a walk.

Practise deep breathing

Deep breathing is a wonderful way to achieve a sense of **calm**. Practise taking slow, deep breaths at least once a day.

The benefits of deep breathing:

- **Your muscles relax**

- **Your blood pressure lowers**

- **Fresh oxygen pours into every cell in the body, improving the efficiency of every system in the body and also leading to physical stamina and greater mental concentration**

- **Endorphins are released, generating feelings of well-being and perhaps also resulting in pain relief**

- **Your lymphatic system works more effectively, helping to rid the body of harmful toxins.**

How to practise deep breathing

1. Lie down in a comfortable, quiet place that is free of distractions

2. Inhale deeply, filling your lungs with air. Bring the air into your abdomen, not just your chest. Count to five as you breathe in

3. Breathe out deeply, emptying your lungs completely. Count again to five as you breathe out. Feel the tension being released from your muscles

4. Continue to inhale and exhale deeply for a few minutes, counting slowly to five each time. Concentrate on only your breathing and counting.

See also the next health tip.

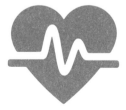

Practise 4-7-8

The 4-7-8 relaxation technique is a powerful variation on deep breathing. It has been shown to slow heart rate, to lower high blood pressure and aid digestion, especially if the exercise is done **twice a day**. The technique can help you cope with stressful situations when you might otherwise feel angry. It can also help quell food and nicotine cravings, and it can be an effective aid for sleeping.

The 4-7-8 technique

1. Start by lightly touching the ridge of tissue behind your top front teeth with your tongue, then exhale completely and do the following breathing pattern

2. Breathe in through your nose quietly for a count of four

3. Hold your breath for a count of seven

4. Blow air out through your mouth for a count of eight, making a *whoosh* sound

5. Repeat the process three more times

6. Do this twice a day

7. After a few weeks' practice, increase the repeat cycle from four to eight breaths each time.

Get a pet

Scientific evidence shows that dog owners tend to be healthier than the average person. A study at Cambridge University found that owning a pet produced improvements in **general health** in as little as one month and this continued over the ten-month study. Pet owners were found to suffer fewer ailments such as headaches, colds and hay fever.

Health benefits from owning a pet, **especially a dog**, include:

- **Dogs are wonderful exercise machines. Unless they're tiny, most dogs need at least a couple of walks a day, which keeps both them and you fitter**

- Stroking a pet or simply watching a fish swim in an aquarium helps you to **relax**. Just watching a pet can reduce heartbeat rate and lower blood pressure

- Research shows that keeping a pet significantly reduces levels of blood cholesterol and triglyceride, two blood fats that can influence heart disease. This may make pet owners less prone to heart attacks. What's more, patients who own a pet have a much better chance of surviving for more than a year after a heart attack – a difference which cannot be explained by the extra exercise that dog owners enjoy

- Children who own pets are often less self-centred

- Psychiatrically ill people are happier as a result of looking after a pet.

Useful websites

Dr Google has become very popular as a health resource for non-medical people. But so much of the information on the internet is of dubious quality, and some of it is not only wrong but frankly dangerous. So here are a few go-to websites that are really trustworthy:

nhs.uk
This has an excellent encyclopaedia of illnesses and a self-diagnosis section that links to quality health information elsewhere including your nearest doctor, dentist, pharmacy and optician.

patient.info
A very user-friendly site with hundreds of information leaflets on health and disease.

nice.org.uk

The website of the Department of Health's National Institute for Clinical Excellence (NICE) has easy-to-read, up-to-date information on a wide range of health conditions and diseases.

bupa.co.uk

Apart from health insurance the site has a really useful A–Z of medical conditions.

surgerydoor.co.uk

Good advice on a wide range of topics. List of remedies for common complaints, and details of their ingredients and approximate cost.

easyhealth.org.uk

A website made so that people know where to find 'accessible' health information. 'Accessible' information is information that uses easy words with pictures.

webmd.boots.com

Provides comprehensive GP-reviewed information and a symptom checker.

healthywomen.org
American one-stop women's health advice. Experts are available to answer questions, and you can read about women with similar concerns.

healthychildren.org
Another excellent American site. Advice on raising your child and also reassurance about medical concerns.

menshealthforum.org.uk
Provides information, services and treatments that men and boys need to live healthier, longer and more fulfilling lives.

thriva.co
Hundreds of reasonably priced blood and other laboratory tests, many via finger-prick blood tests you can do at home, with reports from qualified doctors. Useful when your NHS GP can't or won't arrange a test because of lack of time or funding.

Have you enjoyed this book?

If so, why not write a review on your favourite website?

If you're interested in finding out more about our books,
find us on Facebook at **Summersdale Publishers** and
follow us on Twitter at **@Summersdale**.

Thanks very much for buying this Summersdale book.

www.summersdale.com

Images on p.14, p.21, p.32, p.66, p.78, p.85, p.121, p.157, p.163, p.184 –
© Brothers Good/Shutterstock.com

Images on p.47, p.49, p.51, p.70, p.72, p.93, p.101, p.139, p.166, p.168, p.172, p.174 –
© Design Seed/Shutterstock.com

Image on p.83 – © VectorShop/Shutterstock.com